THINGS THAT GROSS ME OUT!

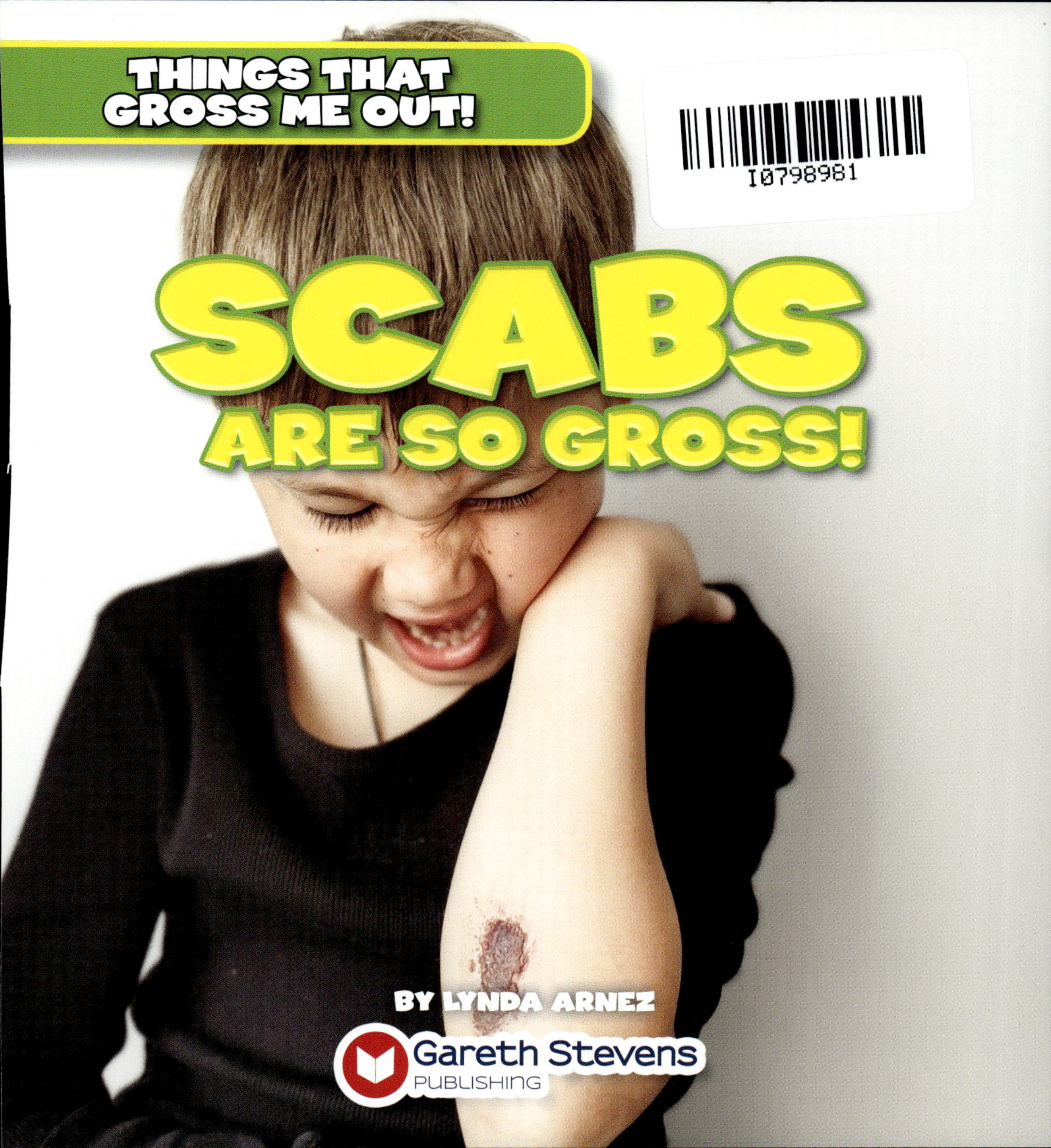

SCABS ARE SO GROSS!

BY LYNDA ARNEZ

Gareth Stevens PUBLISHING

Please visit our website, www.garethstevens.com. For a free color catalog of all our high-quality books, call toll free 1-800-542-2595 or fax 1-877-542-2596.

Cataloging-in-Publication Data

Names: Arnéz, Lynda.
Title: Scabs are so gross! / Lynda Arnéz.
Description: Buffalo, NY : Gareth Stevens Publishing, 2026. | Series: Things that gross me out! | Includes glossary and index.
Identifiers: ISBN 9781482471441 (pbk.) | ISBN 9781482471458 (library bound) | ISBN 9781482471465 (ebook)
Subjects: LCSH: Wounds and injuries–Juvenile literature. | Wound healing–Juvenile literature.
Classification: LCC RD93.A76 2026 | DDC 617.044–dc23

Published in 2026 by
Gareth Stevens Publishing
2544 Clinton Street
Buffalo, NY 14224

Designer: Tanya Dellaccio Keeney
Editor: Kristen Nelson

Photo credits: Cover Sh_olya/Shutterstock.com; p. 5 Aiman Dairabaeva/Shutterstock.com; pp. 7, 9 (illustrations) IGORdeyka/Shutterstock.com; p. 7 (image) Rawpixel.com/Shutterstock.com; p. 9 RINDAWS/Shutterstock.com; p. 11 MagicBones/Shutterstock.com; p. 13 cunaplus/Shutterstock.com; p. 15 Tatevosian Yana/Shutterstock.com; p. 17 Yiorgos GR/Shutterstock.com; p. 19 Alisusha/Shutterstock.com; p. 21 Ermolaev Alexander/Shutterstock.com.

Printed in the United States of America

CONTENTS

Boldface words appear in the glossary.

Ouch!

Have you ever fallen and skinned your knee? How about **scratched** a bug bite so much that it bled? Scabs can form over any place where your skin has been broken. They can look pretty gross!

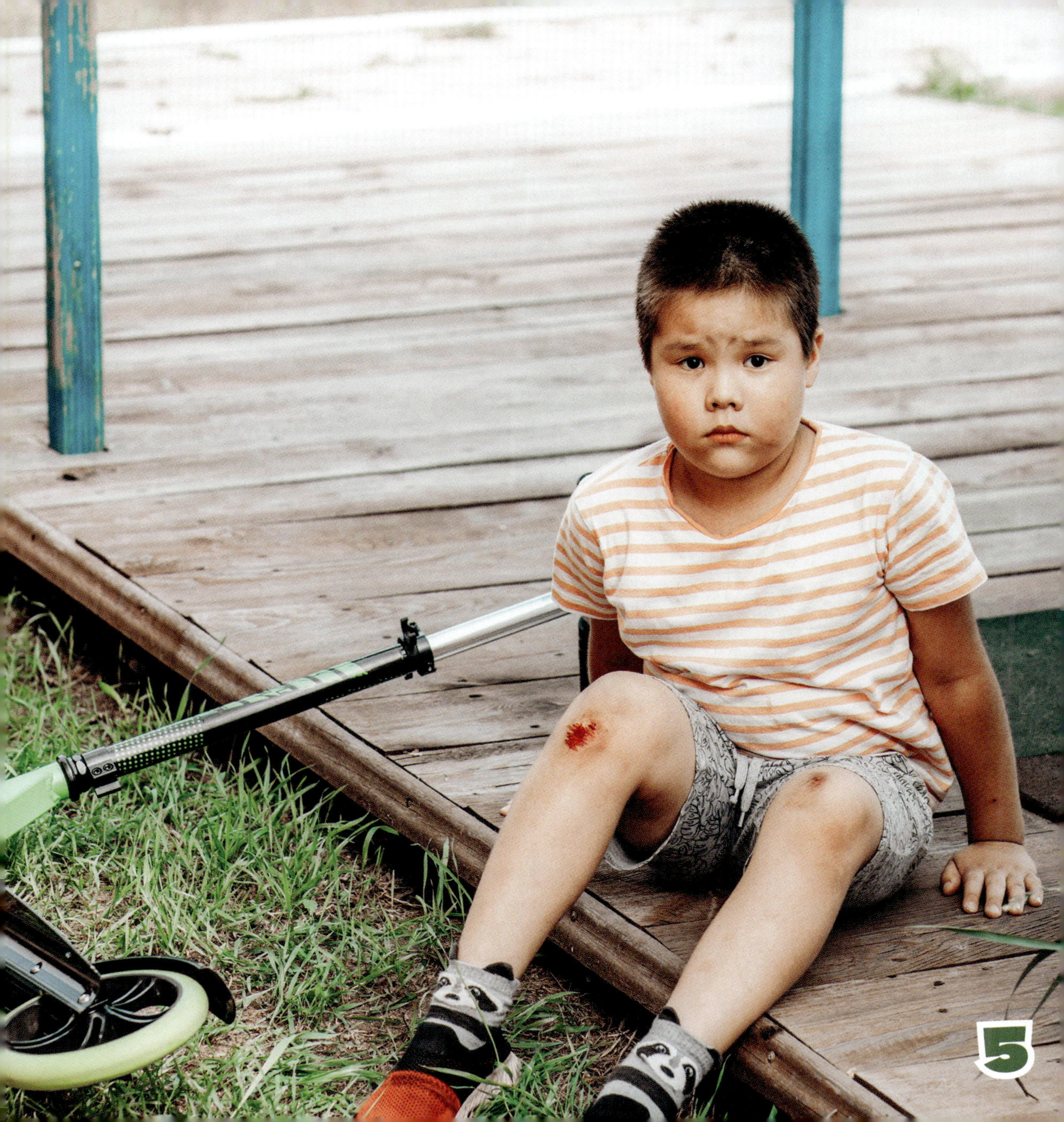

About Blood

After you get a cut or scrape, you may bleed. Your blood is made up of cells. Red blood cells carry **oxygen** around the body. White blood cells help the body fight off illness. The liquid part of blood is called plasma.

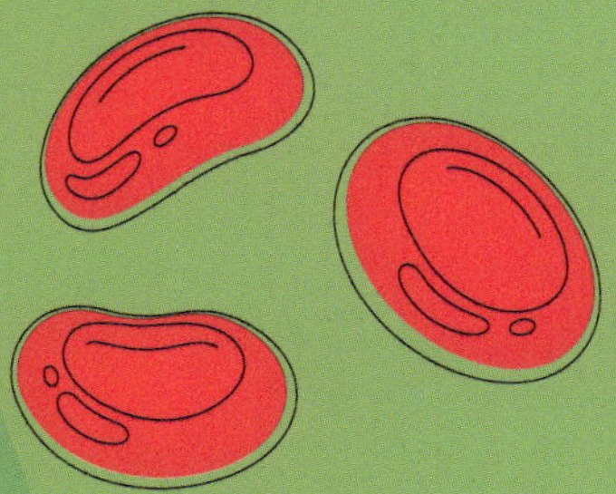

RED BLOOD CELLS

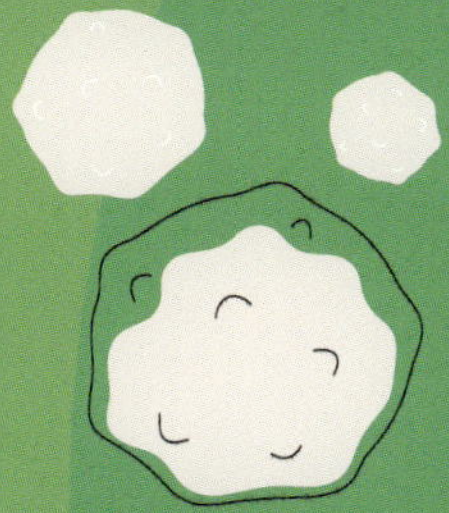

WHITE BLOOD CELLS

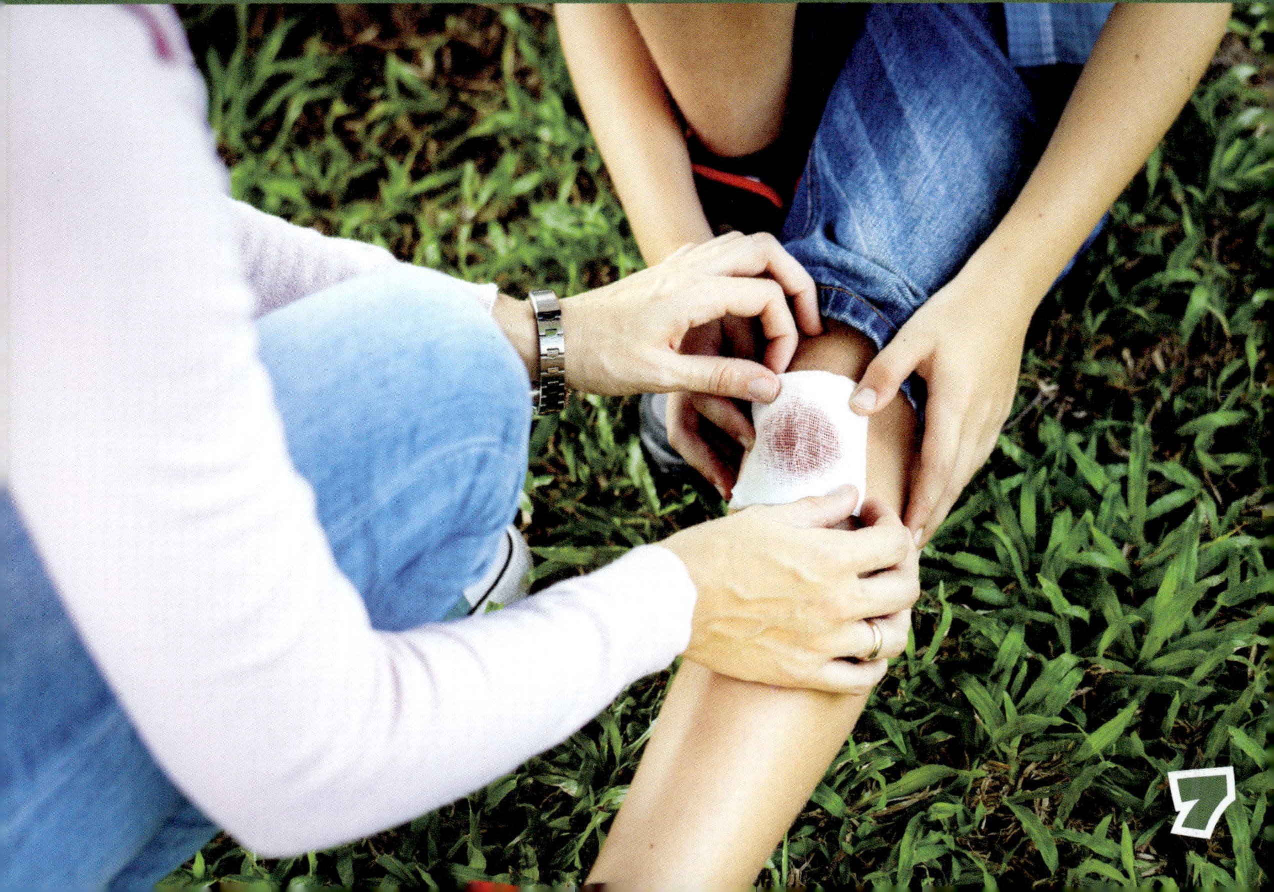

Platelets are parts of the blood that work to stop blood from flowing when you get hurt. This is called clotting. Sticky matter called fibrin, as well as the other kinds of blood cells, hold the clot together.

PLATELETS

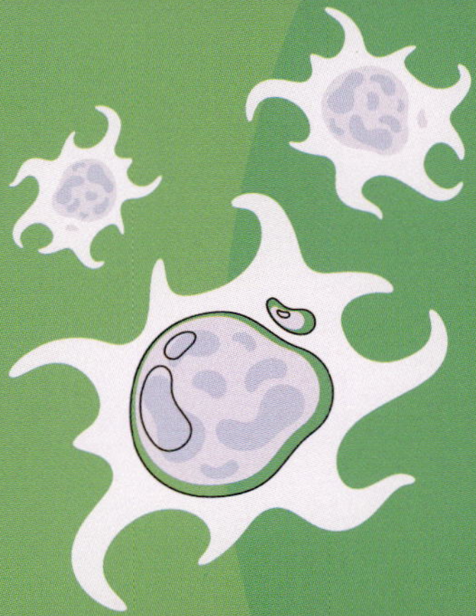

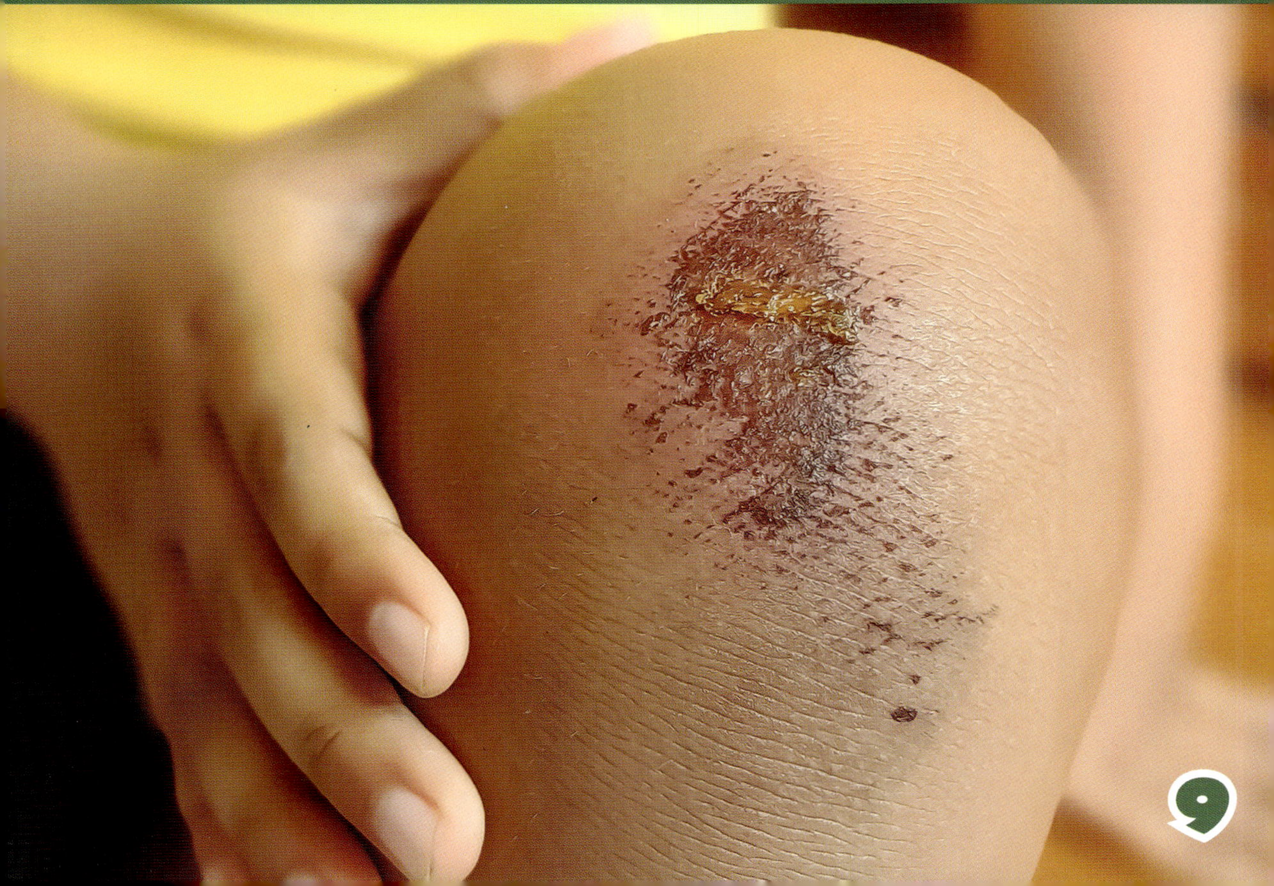

All Dried Up

A scab is the dried-out blood left at the place where you got hurt. It's like a Band-Aid your body makes! Scabs commonly look red or brown. They might feel hard and rough. They may turn white when they get wet.

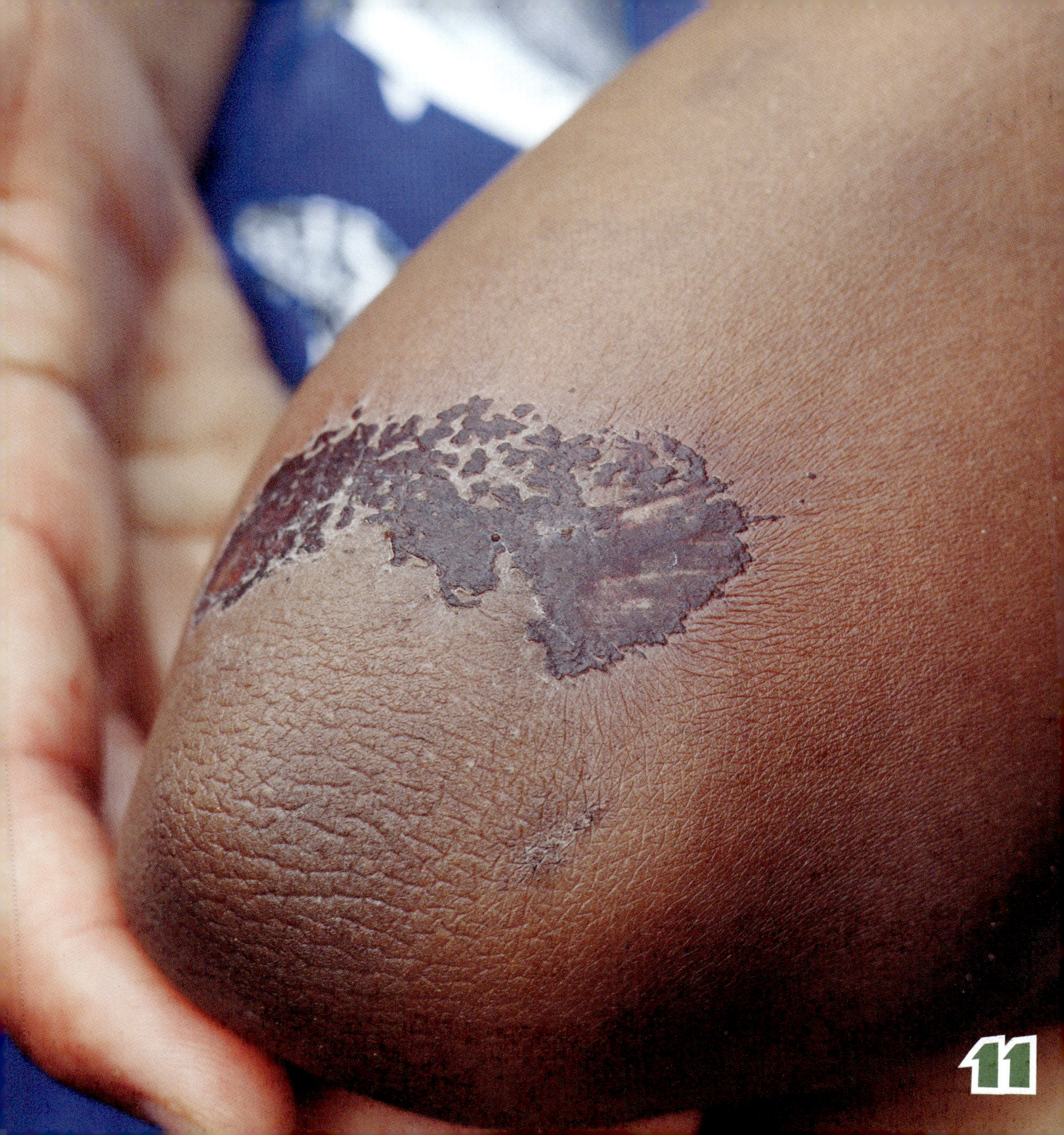

What Scabs Do

Scabs have an important job. First, they stop blood from flowing out of the body. Next, they **protect** the place where the skin has been broken. They keep out germs that could cause an **infection**. They cover the place where the body is regrowing **tissue** like skin.

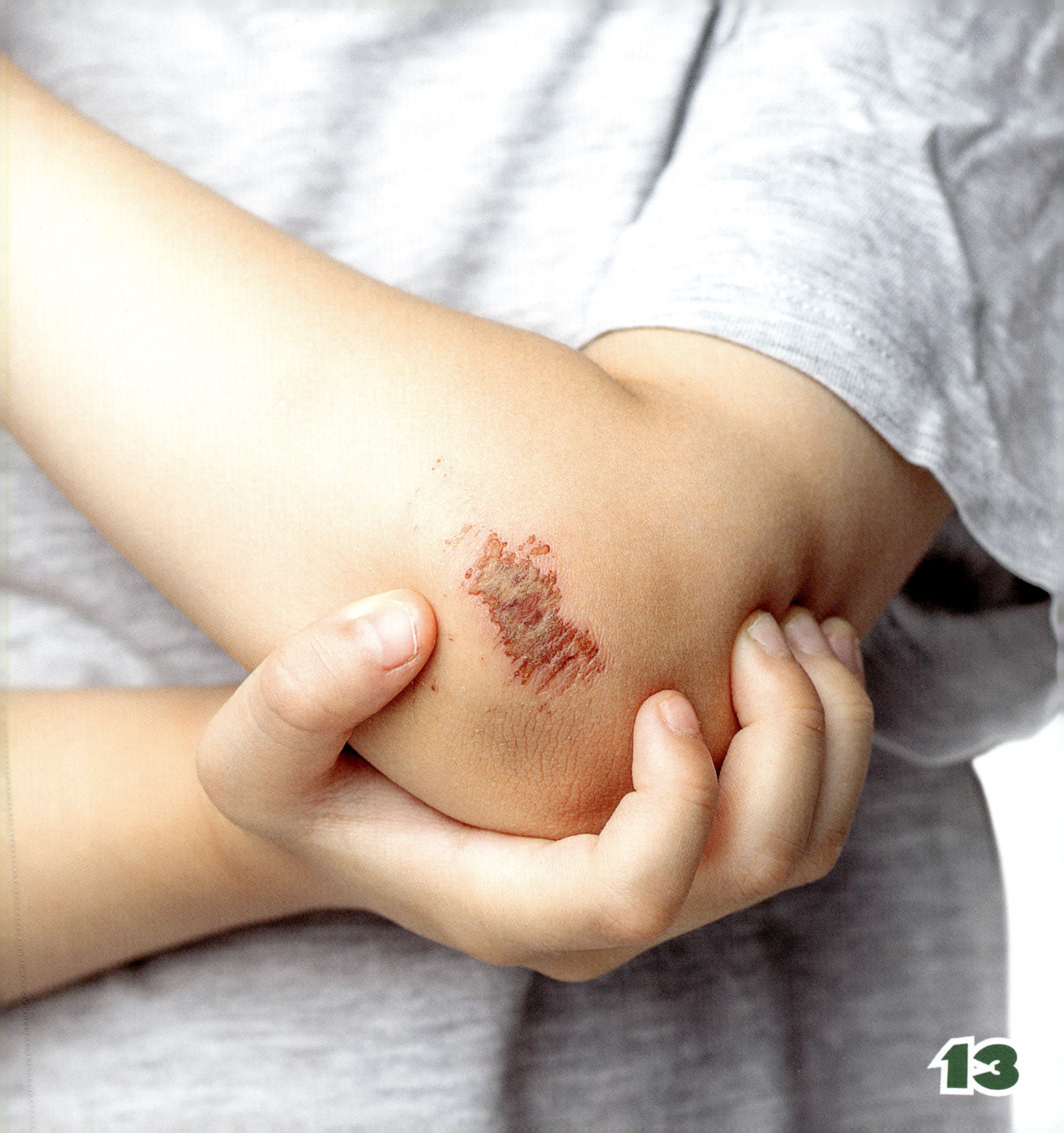

So Itchy!

Scabs **itch**! This is often a sign the body is working to heal. Try not to scratch! Don't pick at your scab either. When a scab comes off too soon, it pulls new tissue cells off. This slows healing.

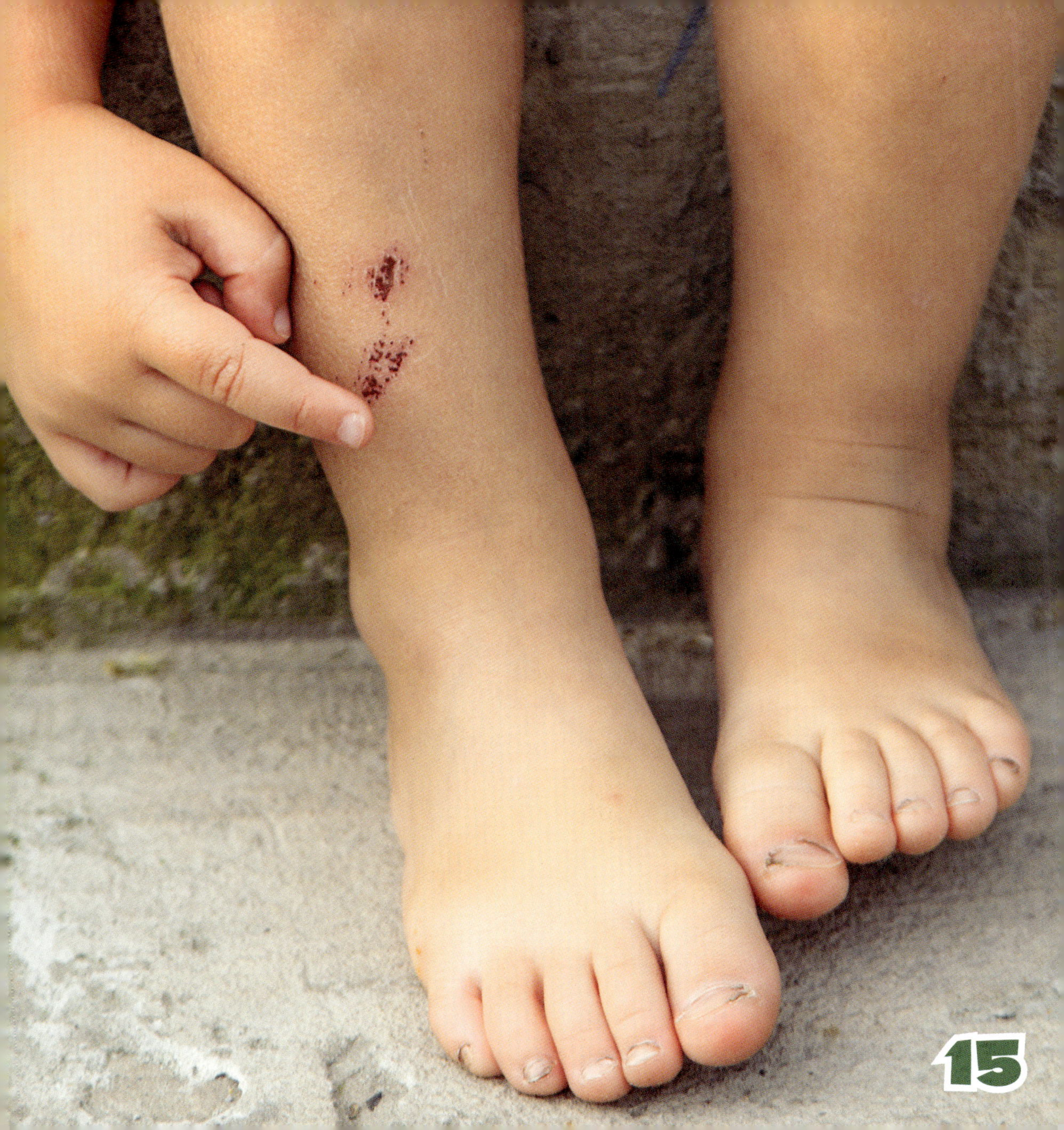

Time to Heal

It takes about a week or two for the scab to heal. The scab will fall off on its own as new skin cells under it grow in. However, the larger the **wound**, the longer this may take. Keeping the scab covered with a bandage can help.

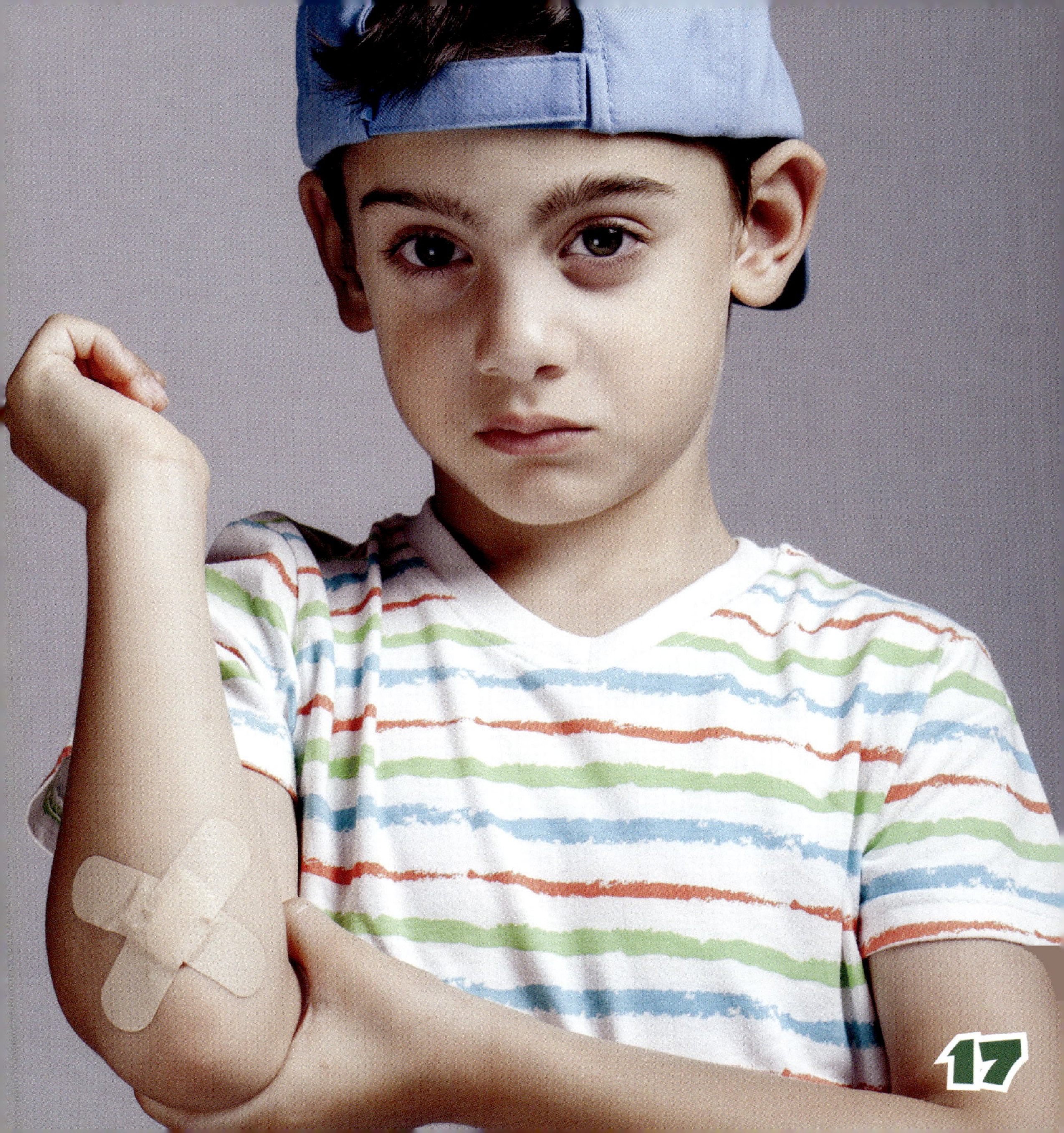

Scab Infections

Keep the area around the scab clean. However, infections can happen. If the scab gets bigger, feels hot, or looks very red, it may be infected. An infected scab can also ooze yellow or green **pus**. Yuck! It's time to see your doctor.

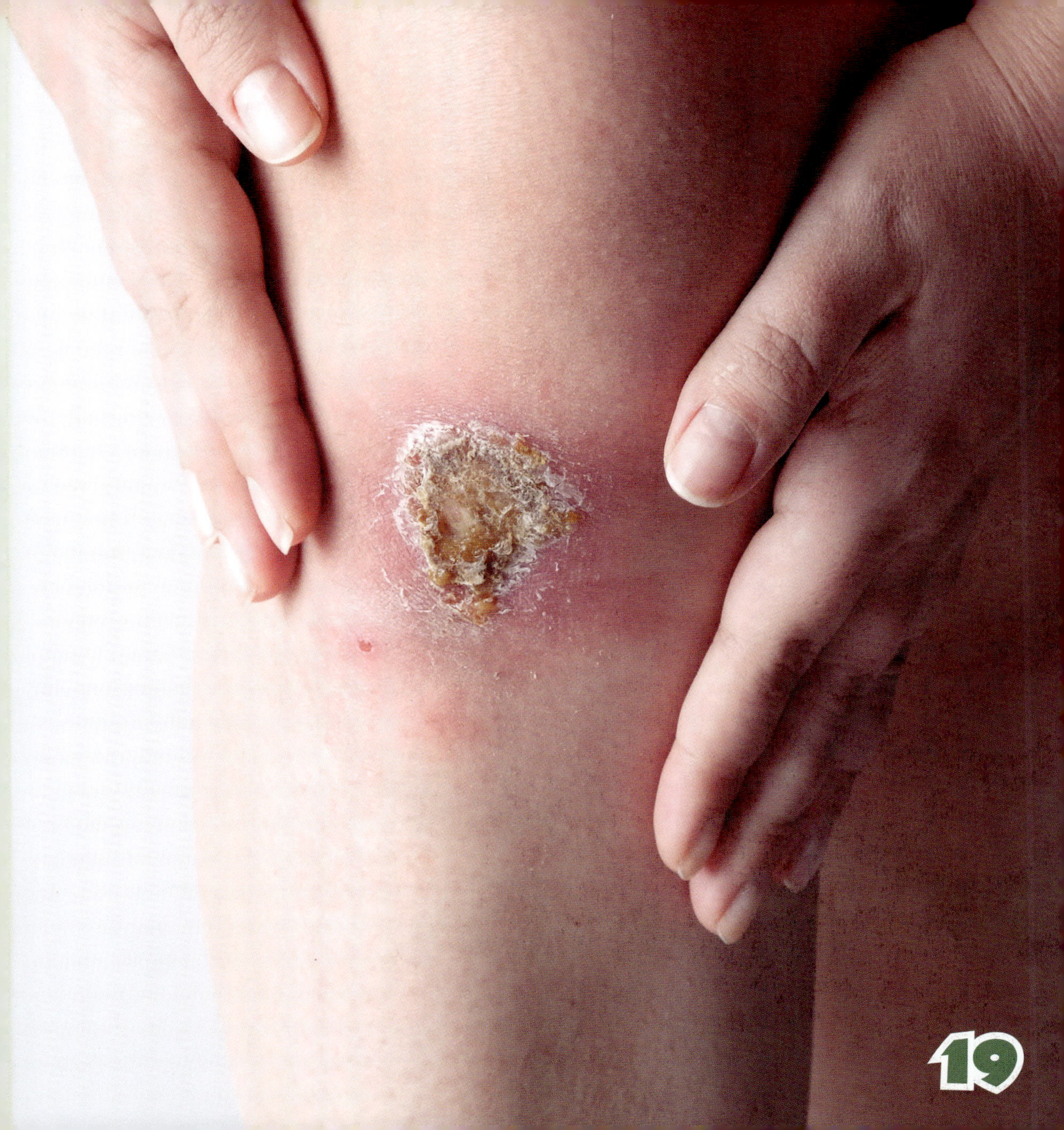

Too Much or Too Little

Some people have **disorders** in which their body does not clot blood well. Instead of a scab, they might just keep bleeding from a cut! There are also disorders in which blood clots inside the body, causing problems.

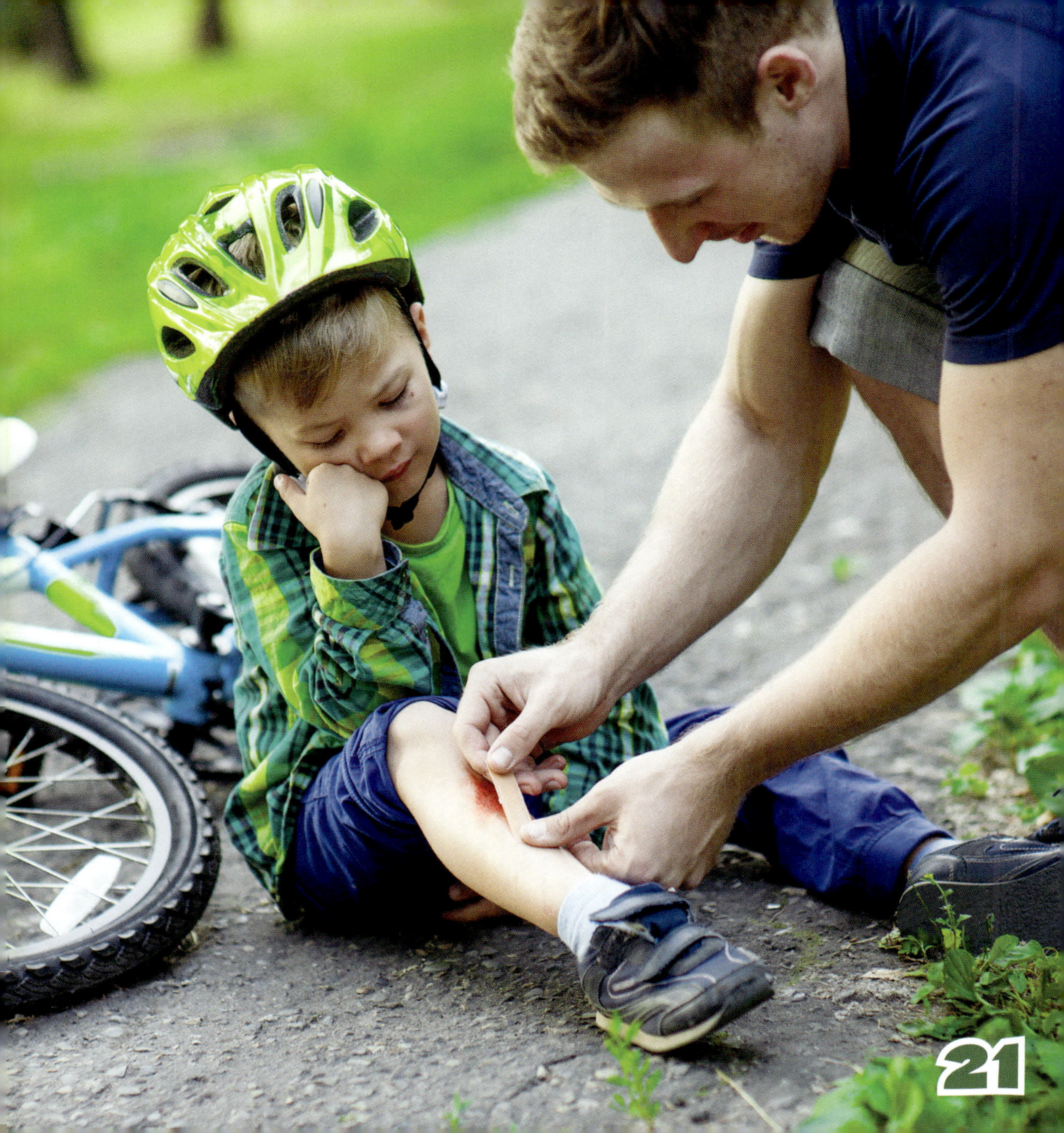

GLOSSARY

disorder: A medical condition that's not usual or normal.

infection: The spread of germs inside the body, causing illness.

itch: To have an unpleasant feeling on your skin that makes you want to scratch.

oxygen: A colorless, odorless gas that many animals, including people, need to breathe.

protect: To keep safe.

pus: Liquid matter that may come out of an infected area.

scratch: To rub or scrape lightly to stop the feeling of an itch.

tissue: Matter that forms the parts of living things.

wound: An injury, like a cut or scrape.

FOR MORE INFORMATION

BOOKS

Branzei, Sylvia. *Nitty-Gritty Grossology: Over 101 Disgusting Facts*. New York, NY: Grosset & Dunlap, 2025.

Jackson, Tom. *The Small and Mighty Book of the Human Body*. London, UK: OH!, an imprint of Welbeck Children's Limited, 2023.

WEBSITES

Stitches
https://kidshealth.org/en/kids/stitches.html
Some cuts need more help! Read about stitches here.

What Are Scabs?
https://kidshealth.org/en/kids/scab.html
Review more information about scabs for kids.

Publisher's note to educators and parents: Our editors have carefully reviewed these websites to ensure that they are suitable for students. Many websites change frequently, however, and we cannot guarantee that a site's future contents will continue to meet our high standards of quality and educational value. Be advised that students should be closely supervised whenever they access the internet.

INDEX